Dedication

To everyone who wants to improve their sex-life

Table of Contents

Chapter 1:

Erectile dysfunction -What and Why?

We all are well aware and willing to discuss our health problems so that we remain in good physical form. Unfortunately, when it comes to our sexual performance / health we hardly tend to open up about the dysfunctions and irregularities. Nevertheless, they hamper our sexual life to such extent which may be irreparable. It's well known that people suffering from such disorders develop an inferiority complex which often becomes the cause of other psychological and mental problems.

I wish to reach to my readers that there should be no shying away from this issue. WE should treat this challenge no different than the other diseases like obesity, diabetes. In my opinion, longer we hesitate in fixing this problem, the stronger it becomes. People with this challenge remain unknown, just because people don't accept the fact that they have the sexual disorder. My advice - forget about your ego for a moment and start doing something about this. Buying this book is the first step.

Fortunately, Erectile Dysfunction is not just treatable, but also curable. Although, to get rid of it completely you have to address the underlying cause of the problem first. People don't like to admit it, but the primary cause of Erectile Dysfunction is because of the lifestyle you've chosen. You won't be able to cure this problem if you're not ready to make changes in your life.

Many people think that these disorders pass on from one generation to another, or they symbolize a lack of libido. These thoughts are nothing more than the crap that keeps them away from coming out with the problem. They don't even believe that there's a cure. Thankfully, they're mistaken.

There are a lot of cases reported and yet the number awaits to triple fold if the private ones are also considered. Another thing to keep settle with is nothing is without cause if it happened to you it has a reason. Let's have a quick look at the possible causes that paves a way to this highly uninvited circumstance.

Now it has been proven that male sexual excitements are a compiled process involving several factors like brain, hormones, emotions, nerves, muscles and blood vessels. When so many aspects influence the sexual arousal in men, then they can obviously be hindered by any. But the most foreseen among them is stress or bad mental health as per reports is believed. Stress not only causes erectile dysfunction but at times worsen it to a highly dangerous level.

Very often psychological and physical issues have a combined result in a form of sexual dysfunction. For example, if someone has been suffering from any physical pain that slows down sexual response may develop a kind of mental pressure blended with anxiety to hold an erection. In my opinion, anxiety is the main evil-doer of sexual dysfunction. Other psychological problems are spoiling the condition at its worst. It draws you to a never-ending cycle when a male fails to perform sexually the atmosphere in the relationship gets soured at some point which puts you in a state of depression.

There are few listed diseases which are more than often responsible for this male sexual disorder. They are low testosterone, clogged blood vessels, diabetes, high cholesterols, obesity, heart disease, multiple sclerosis and Parkinson's disease. The other could be alcoholism, smoking, drug addiction, and tobacco. Having a healthy body matters. Certain medications for the treatment of prostate cancer and surgeries of pelvic areas or spinal cord are also the causes of ED. There's one factor working in our favor - when we know the cause, curing it will not be a problem. I'll talk about that more in-depth in Chapter 4.

Losing the ability to obtain an erection is the biggest fear in men's life. Thank You for taking the first step towards improving your sexual life and therefore – improving your life in general.

Chapter 2:

Recognize the problem.

"The first step in solving a problem is to recognize that it does exist."

- Zig Ziglar

Treatment of any disease depends on two factors, but a first thing is recognizing the problem. Now when we know there could be more than one reason behind erectile dysfunction it's naturally expected that symptoms should vary depending upon the cause. So the problem is said to have abilities to manifest it in many ways. There's a reason you clicked on this book.

Even if you don't have ED or if You don't want to admit it – you'll find the advice in this book very beneficial to your sexual health.

There nothing to lose, but everything to gain.

If it happens more or less transient or momentarily, there is nothing to worry about. Nearly all men face this at some point in their lives, but it is not a big deal and certainly you should not take much stress about it. Similarly is the dysfunction shows a gradual development and then seems to persist, you need to face it. In these conditions, it is typically seen that physical reason is behind it and is called chronic impotence.

An erection problem when to get associated with pain then it's something more serious, the disease is called Peyronie's disease. The erectile dysfunction can be symptoms of other. When your mind indicates that there are any of the listed symptoms, don't waste time just run to the doctor. It's for your good and in the long run, could even prove vital to save your relationship.

Chapter 3:

Why ED is Dangerous

More or less, each and every disorder has its side effects with fewer exceptions. But the astonishing fact remains that even their treatments have some effects that are not needed in our body. ED is a serious sexual health issue so it certainly won't be life threatening or pose other physical problems. On the other hand, it affects adversely on our mental status. It leads us to low self-esteem and depression due to the soured relationship when a person fails to perform during intercourse. And we all know that having low self-esteem and being in a depressive state will cause other problems, that's why it's crucial to deal with it.

Look its treatments have more complicated health issues on one's body at a physical level than the disease itself. For example, Viagra is a drug used in its medication contains phosphodiesterase inhibitors. First and foremost warning, PDE should not be used by men who take medicine containing nitrates which are used to treat angina. Blood thinning medicine users, enlarged prostate and high BP patients should also keep caution rather take extra care with ED pills. These issues should be discussed with your physician before starting treatment for erectile dysfunction. One more thing to remember, when PDE and these drugs interact they automatically pave a way for physical agonies like a headache, nasal congestion, upset stomach plus hearing and vision problems.

A history of heart disease, uncontrolled diabetes, past or recent strokes and extremely low or very high BP patients are also advised to discuss the side effects of such treatments before starting it with their doctors in length. It is imperative for the complete well-being of your own body. After all, we don't want to cure a disease and get two more in return.

Your body is Your temple. Take a good care of it.

Chapter 4:

Causes of Erectile Dysfunction

As I already mentioned in the first Chapter, there are many causes of Erectile Dysfunction. Most of us are embarrassed to visit a doctor and talk about of disorder. We hope for a simple and instant cure in for of pill. Often, a doctor will ask for a complete diagnosis to ensure that there are no serious health problems. ED doesn't come alone. It happens for a reason – there's something wrong with your physical or mental health.

The way we chose to lead our lives have direct effects on our health and body. They are directive guidelines to what our body will be going through. A healthy lifestyle undoubtedly will positively impact on our body. This particular theory goes round the similar way, so it's but natural that unhealthy lifestyle habits are going to bring something or other unwanted situation related to our overall well-being. It has been discovered that erectile dysfunction is caused or worsened in many men due to their wrong lifestyle choices. In my practice, undoing them could help a lot in the whole process of recovery.

There are main lifestyle factors and health conditions that are causing your dysfunction.

Obesity

You'll notice that adding a few more extra pounds will not only change your physique but also change your state of mind. Being obese makes you sick, sad and depressed. Having a high body-fat percentage will cause Erectile Dysfunction. Your body will start to slow the production of testosterone. But increase production of estrogen, a female sex hormone. You'll find it difficult to maintain an erection. There's a rumor that fat men last longer, but I totally disagree with that.

Diabetes

Can be caused by obesity and will negatively affect your whole body. It will elevate your sugar levels, men with diabetes have damaged nerves and different blood vessel problems, this means having erection problems is inevitable. Men with diabetes don't have problems with libido. Unfortunately, they're usually not hard enough for penetration or are not able to get an erection.

Heart Disease

A bad diet and lifestyle often lead to the hardening of your arteries as plaques form around the blood vessel, and it causes blood vessels to narrow, making it difficult for blood to pass through them. Usually, smaller blood vessels get affected first – the blood vessels leading to the penis. There is the reason why doctors very often see

ED as an early sign of plaque appearance in the blood vessels. If you do not treat this problem, it might as well be fatal.

Pornography

I've decided to put this very high on the risk because there are too many men who still watch pornography while being in the relationships. It not only drains your energy, affects your mentally and also lowers your libido. I've also suffered because of the pornography, and I got problems getting excited by real sexual encounters. I challenge you do stop watching porn for a month. You'll even see the difference in your sex life within the first two weeks.

Smoking

Here's another reason to quit smoking, just by saying "no" to the cigarette will help you to achieve firmer, harder, thicker and longer erections. The problems here is – Smoking damages your blood vessels and interferes with blood flow. However, you might not realize how big of an impact cigarette has on your body. Thankfully, smoking does not cause extensive damage to your body. That does not apply if you've been smoking for the past few years, having a cigarette few times per month is totally okay.

Your penis and Your body will be grateful, when You quit inhaling the cigarette.

Alcoholism

Another common cause of Erectile Dysfunction, it could cause temporary problems, but can eventually lead to a long-term condition. And again, alcohol reduces blood flow not only to the brain but your penis as well. Men who drink alcohol tend to have a weaker orgasm, lack of sexual desire and premature ejaculation. My advice on alcohol – drink only the best quality alcohol only and in moderation. A day after drinking you should cleanse your body, by drinking at least 4 liters of water.

Processed or low-quality Foods

The American diet is filled with trans*fats, different preservatives, GMO foods and contain a lot of sugars. That's why we have young guys in their early 20's with Erectile Dysfunction. It's all over the internet; transfats are the cause of different disorders, such as ED and obesity. Your body is unhealthy and weak on the inside. Your body is too busy removing all the junk; that 's why procreative ability has to suffer.

Medications

Many drugs could cause Erectile Dysfunction. For example Antidepressants (Prozac, for instance), many different Cholesterol Lowering Drugs, Heartburn Medications. You should do your research on this. Experts say that many different medications affect your hormones and neurotransmitters. Stick to natural remedies if you can.

Chapter 5:

Natural Cures for Erectile Dysfunction

The best part of this book. Thankfully, Erectile Dysfunction is curable and reversible. You're probably suffering this conditions because of health and lifestyle. In my opinion, your penis shows what's happening in the rest of the body. It displays the lack of balance between mind and body. When you get your health and life in balance, things will go smooth again. The sad news is, you'll have to make changes to your lifestyle.

Healthy Eating

Unfortunately, there's no such thing as a "magic food" that grants you vigorous and instant erections if you consume it in large quantity. In my experience, changing the quality of your food at least for one week will make you feel entirely different. Keep your food consumption balance and emphasize on healthy, organic food items, while avoiding processed and low-quality foods.

What should you eat?

Fruits – all fruits will be great for your body, but you'd want to choose ones high in vitamin C. Studies show, that regular consumption of vitamin C will drastically improve your sperm quality.

Green veggies – including lettuce, cabbage, spinach and more. Spinach contains large quantities of magnesium which will help with the dilation of blood vessels. Spinach is also rich in folate – substance that is linked to the prevention of plaque buildup in your blood vessels. They help with blood circulations, meaning, you'll have harder erections. I always eat 50g-100g of spinach a day. Add then to your salad!

Eggs – high in protein and contain many vitamins, eggs can help with weight loss. They balance hormones in your body and can boost the level of libido, regardless if you're male or female. My father in law drinks five quail eggs every day (they do not contain salmonella, so you can use them raw) and always says that only because of this food he can have "erection like 20 years old" he's at his late 50. As from my experience, these eggs drastically increase my libido. They are high in cholesterol, which will help with testosterone production. I strongly suggest you do use five quail eggs every day for a least a month; you 'll feel the difference.

Fish – fatty fish is good for you, not only because it has omega-3 fatty acids, but also because of the high contents of L-arginine – compound that boosts hormone production. Also, you should supplement with high-quality fish oil.

Dark Chocolate – There's a recent study found that flavonoids in dark chocolate can improve circulation. That could be useful for erection problems that are due to poor circulation. Flavonoids are natural- occurring antioxidants that protect plants from toxins and help repair cell damage. Studies show that flavonoids and other antioxidants have similar effects on people. They may help lower blood pressure and decrease cholesterol, both of which are factors that contribute to erectile dysfunction. The sad thing is, most chocolate in the market is filled with many different preservatives.

Other foods – Red meat, grass fed. Too much red meat could be bad for you. Nuts, peanuts are an excellent source of healthy fats. A study found that men with erectile dysfunction who consumed pistachio nuts every day for three weeks experienced significant improvement in sexual issues, including ED, sexual desire, and overall sexual satisfaction. Berries, fresh berries are one of the most powerful disease-fighting foods available, filled with many natural antioxidants.

Chapter 6:

Weight Lifting and Weight Loss

As a certified personal trainer, I've different opinion, unlike the most authors who write about this. They are not giving the best quality advice and sometimes their advice does more harm than good. Please understand, everything written is this book is critical, one change to your lifestyle won't fix your condition. But the weight-lifting and exercising is the most impactful. After this book, I'll be releasing more in-depth guide about exercising.

The effects of exercise on people with ED are awesome. For individuals who are obese / overweight, using not only will burn few pounds, but also decrease the chance of having heart disease and diabetes – also linked to Erectile Dysfunction.

If you're already at your ideal weight and have a healthy body-fat percentage, it's still a good idea to do different exercises, just to maintain your physique or boost your self-esteem. When you're confident about your looks, you'll have fewer inhibitions in bed; that will result in more satisfying sex and intimacy with your partner. Exercising will improve your whole physique and treat any other health problem that you might have. Exercising will boost oxygen in the body, improve circulation of the blood and increase production of nitric oxide within your body. The reason you get strong erections while being on Viagra is because of the nitric oxide. There's no need to use a blue pill; you can get the same effect naturally.

It's well known, that testosterone, a male sex hormone has an enormous impact on a man's reproductive and sexual function. The best way to boost your T-levels naturally is to do weight-lifting. Lower the number of reps and increase the weight. If you've been doing bodybuilding type routines all the time, heavy weight-lifting will also break plateau effect, and you'll get more results.

Stick to the compound exercises that work for large muscle groups, for example, squats, deadlifts. Yes, I knew they're painful, but the reward is huge. You should ideally be using 80-95% of your 1RM (one rep max). Your goal should be 5-8 reps for 2-5 sets. Aim for 2-3 weight-lifting workouts per week, supplemented with 1-2 days of cardio. Studies have shown that HIIT training, bicycling, boxing, running can increase production of hormones and improve your mental health. Although, if you're a beginner, I strongly recommend you to hire a personal trainer. There are a lot of young guys who would work with you for a low price, just to gain experience. Forget about your ego.

Chapter 7:

Quit Smoking

First and foremost thing quit smoking! If you have trouble quitting, try some professional help. Nicotine replacement like gum and lozenges would help you to get rid of the unhealthy habit. This step is quite recommendable for the complete goodness of your health and immunity. Let's be honest here, quitting smoking is not an easy job, but it's well-known about how much cigarette affects your body and sexual health. Is it worth it?

This book is not about smoking, but I'll give you a template on how you should approach it. Before we start, I would like to guess why most people are smoking.

Process. You probably love the process of it. Putting the cigarette in your mouth, lighting in up and feeling instant gratification. I'll ask again, is it worth it? The reward of not smoking is too high. You're using external and unnatural methods to feel relaxed, and what do you expect? You get an unnatural response from your body, in a form of ED. Your body punishes you because you harm it with your actions. If you love the process that much, there are a lot of techniques that you can use to feel relaxed. I could write a book about it, do your research on this. Alternatively, you could use E-cigarette without preservatives and nicotine. I haven't used this personally, but my friends had a magnificent success with it.

People around You. Probably your co-worker, family members, and friends are also smoking, and you go "with the flow" and have smoke with them, just to feel closer to them. And when you say that you're quitting the cigarette they laugh at you or look at you in disbelief. They will try to affect you and your decision of quitting the nicotine. That's because they want to drag you down to their level. They don't want you to surpass them because it will show the weakness it themselves. Let's the honest, if you quit smoking that already indicates that you have more self-discipline and a stronger will-power than other smokers you know. Do your own conclusions. Period.

• Decide on a day you quit smoking.

• A week or two weeks before that day lower your consumption of nicotine.

• Fight the craving.

• Reward yourself for EACH day of resisting the temptation. Remember the quote, *What gets rewarded, gets repeated.*

• A healthy body already is a reward. A reward that money can't buy. But we all live in the material world, buy yourself a snack or go to the movies. It's up to you.

• Decide on a **punishment.** If you failed, you deserve to be punished. Decide on your own.

• Have an accountability partner. There's nothing wrong to ask for help. Just find a person who truly cares about you and your health.

Your accountability can't be a smoker for obvious reasons.

• Have smoke once in a while. I usually smoke a cigar once per month just to relax even more. This way, I'm NOT being used by a substance, but using it myself. I'm in control, but smokers – are not, that's why they can't quit smoking. Period.

Chapter 8:

What Should You NOT Do

Processed and Fried Food Choices

That also means quitting fast-food, this includes hot dogs, sausages, bacon, burgers or anything else unhealthy. You'll find that these foods contain a very high amount of salt, sugar, preservatives and low-quality carbohydrates. Yes, processed food is much cheaper than organic and healthy food, it's made on purpose. You should ask yourself is your health and well-being more important than a piece of paper. Note: I strongly suggest you to stop using vegetable oils, I use coconut oil or best quality olive oil. There are many different health benefits, just by consuming one teaspoon of coconut oil before breakfast will make a big difference.

Alcohol Consumption

Let's be honest; alcohol is a depressant, it can decrease your sexual desire, make you depressed, make it hard to achieve an erection. The entirely different effect can be accomplished if it's used in moderation. Moderation is the key; the same things are with smoking – you have to be in control. I'll even further, you suffer them Erectile Dysfunction because YOU'RE NOT IN CONTROL. If you are not able to control your life, then how do you expect to control your penis? Don't get offended. You'll not read anything like this in other books – other authors don't want to help you.

Sleep

Sleep deprivation is torture for your body, and it pushes person's psychological and mental well-being the edge. Being tired will not make you want to have sex, you might be ready mentally, but your body will be drained, you'll have difficulty attaining an erection. Note: if you're experimenting with polyphasic sleep schedule, make sure that you're healthy enough. Meaning, your nutrition, lifestyle have to be balanced.

Here's some techniques you can use to have a better sleep:

• Avoid computers, TV, mobile phone an hour before sleep.

• Don't drink coffee 4 hours before bed.

• Listen to audiobook or read a book in your bed.

• Make sure your room is *completely dark,* only exception is candle light.

• Don't eat too much before bed.

• Based on my experience, protein and fats will help you to fall asleep faster. I usually start and end my day with fat/protein meals. *Why do you need carbs in your sleep?*

Chapter 9:

Herbs and Supplements

Many herbs and supplements will help you with your condition. Not only good for your sexual health, but also for your overall health. I suggest to use them in the purest form because you might never know how other preservatives could affect you. If a label is too fancy – don't buy it. Don't buy overpriced supplements – there isn't much of a difference. You could save even more money by purchasing directly from the manufacturer. Without the further due, let's continue.

L - Arginine

Very useful amino acid, especially if you're going to the gym. It helps with blood circulatory problems, regulates blood pressure and prevents heart disease. Your body needs a little help because it doesn't pump enough blood into your penis, that's why you experience no erection. This amino acid is in foods such as pumpkin seeds, peanuts, walnuts. Also Garlic help with blood flow. I eat a lot of garlic with my foods; that 's why I don't use salt, ketchup or anything else.

Horny Goat Weed

It is an extremely legit herb. This substance is always used in Testosterone boosters and other "Man's Health" related supplements. Horny goat weed will give you similar effect that Viagra does. Just don't overuse it. It's very cheap and available everywhere. From my experience – use it 5 hours before sex.

Hawthorn Berry and Cayenne

Both will help you with blood circulation and will make you **extra hard.** I still sometimes buy these, just to give my woman even more pleasure. Very easy to buy online and is available in capsules. **Do not overuse.**

Disclaimer: I'm not a doctor. Consult with the doctor about how these substances could affect your health. What works for me, might not work for you.

Chapter 10:

Conclusion

In the end, I'll tell you that Erectile Dysfunction is easy to stay away from. All you need is awareness and understanding that it is just another disease which you can deal with quickly. Besides it is also relatively rare to get entangled in the web of ED once you have been out of the situation. Your doctor will make sure from his side but do your bit too for a healthy lifestyle. Although, it's up to you to conquer this challenge. **If I could do that, so can YOU! I have total faith in You!**

Good luck my friends!

Book on Porn Addiction

Chapter 1:

Foreword

The idea of a full pair of breasts or a well-toned backside can drive millions of people insane with need. The mere thought of enjoying such sexualized visions can push people into a frenzy. Driving them to obsess compulsively over the sexual ideas attached to the human form. Addiction is a mental and behavioral disorder.

Pornography addiction is a hotly argued and contested disease. The definition of the ailment is compulsive, repeated use of pornographic material until it causes serious negative consequences to the individual's physical, mental, social or financial well-being. This controversial topic is part of the great debate as to its actual existence.

In an age where the internet and unlimited cable offer an instantaneous glimpse into the world of porn how much is too much? The one click society has a smorgasbord of opportunity to enjoy pornography in varied mediums. Hiding nudie magazines under your bed is no longer the way that people enjoy their proclivities in private.

Pornography has been around since prehistoric times. Early rock art evolved into rock and marble figurines, which then became rich oils and beautiful drawings. No matter your personal view on the topic, the impact of capturing human's sexual fantasies in art and literature cannot be denied. To some it is art and to others, it is a vulgar display of actions that should be kept private and discreet.

The advent of printing and then video only compounded the need and, therefore, addiction of the public. With the first laws on the subject of pornography instituted as early as 1857, it has become a taboo and even evil topic to some. Still, the need for it has only grown with time and availability. The public's perception of the idea of Pornography Addiction also seems to waver. Some feel it a victimless disease or crime; with only the individual being affected. Others still believe that the people involved in the "business" of pornography are being used and in some cases abused.

Pornography addiction wasn't even considered by the medical field until recently. The first peer review was only published in 2014. Until that point, it had been taken into account a bad habit by most, with the adage "boys being boys" fitting the attitude towards the problem. Most studies up to that point had been focused on the cultural impact and its effect on feminism.

Still, the problem is real. The pornography industry is a billion dollar cash cow. Take for example that in 1970 the retail totals for porn in America was approximately 10 million dollars. Jump to 1998 and the totals are estimated to be between 750 million to 1 billion dollars. Of course, the estimated totals of $2.6 to $3.9 in 2001 should not surprise anyone.

Pornography is everywhere. So the increase in public consumption is not to be denied. The increase in availability has spawned a more varied and specific demand for the material. There are now specialized types of pornography know as fetish porn. From straight, gay and lesbian porn all the way to the animal enthusiasts and costume junkies; there is a niche for everyone.

Some may believe that the more that is offered, the bigger the demand continues to become. However, that may not necessarily be true. The increase in availability may have just allowed for those with hidden addictions to become more open about their desires. Still, the question remains; is pornography addiction a real problem?

Chapter 2:

Introduction

The main purpose of this book is not to assist you to end masturbating or cut it off entirely, ejaculating and masturbating are normal biological mechanisms. This one should not be ashamed of any matter what, the purpose of the book is to address pornography and the effects it has on your life on a deep subconscious level and how to prevent it from taking over you.

I've struggled with addiction to pornography for about five years. I have tried and attempted to break free countless of times to no avail, and I know how it's like to want to quit something badly yet still fall back into bad habits!
I very well know the frustration, the hurt and the pain, the feeling of unworthiness and the sense of having no control whatsoever. Luckily for you, I've experienced and tested out many techniques and in this, I will be laying an excellent foundation that will aid you in your journey of breaking free and starting a new life.

This book will mainly help you:

1) Understanding why you're wired to keep falling into this habit.

2) Understanding the truth behind the porn industry.

3) Forming new habits that will last long and help you reach the outcome you desire.

4) Understanding the consequences of not breaking free and taking action.

Chapter 3:

Porn Industry – The Truth

Don't underestimate the industry; you are not just getting pleasure, you're getting hooked so that you'd generate them tons of cash profits by countlessly browsing videos and coming across ads.

 They sell you the idea of perfect bodies and shapes while most of the pornstars undergo countless surgeries, I mean come on it's their profession (fake breasts, asses, tons of makeup, perfect filming from certain angles, etc...).

How does this affect you? Just by merely watching this you'll start feeling insecure about your body and the shame behind this will drive you to play it safe and avoid looking for a potential partner.

Even worse, if you ever find a great potential partner, you'll be judging them based on the standards you've seen and inculcated into your mind from hours and hours of browsing the web.

Arousal issues and problems.

If you watch porn regularly, then you'd know how difficult it is to get turned on without it.

It'll be extremely difficult for you to get aroused and just try imagining the shame of not getting excited in real life.

Pornography will cause you difficulties getting aroused in real time since you're hardwired to surfing for at least 20 minutes before deciding it's time, it's hard to fool your brain, it'll crave for the variety you always experience before getting aroused since you've made it a habit.

The crazy blowjob and orgies you get to watch are far from what you want.

Sex is an expression mechanism of love and willingness to spend a lifetime with somebody.

Most of us are looking for a real relationship based on understanding and respect, even if you find yourself denying it, deep down inside it's a need rooted in your nervous system. Most people are genuinely disturbed by blowjobs and orgies. .

Would you want to share your wife/husband with another person? I highly doubt it.

It destroys your moral code of how you treat women / men and relationships. Do not underestimate this, pornography depicts genders as lustful and treats them as objects to charm your sexual energy with no value to personal integrity.

One night stands may be fun, but they certainly do not fill that gap which you're trying to seal shut, human beings are driven towards intimacy and fulfilling relationships, it's a survival mechanism carved and hardwired into our brains. You're being taught to confuse reality for illusion; it 's like expecting a unicorn when watching a horse giving birth, and it's never going to happen no matter how many horse births you watch.

You just have to stop cheating yourself and allow yourself to experience the world as it is cause your world is a reflection of your thoughts and values, believe me, with the right habits and values it'll be worth it. So worthy that one day you're going to look back and disbelieve having watched this crap for so long.

Chapter 4:

Important Things to Understand

Porn feels great at first when you start indulging in it only to find later on that it captivated your mind and shackled you to the iron bars of helplessness.

When you first get started, you experience massive amounts of pleasure looking at naked bodies of the other gender, imagining yourself there scoring and trying to immerse yourself in the experience of imagining yourself there experiencing the orgasm.

So far so good, right?

What you don't realize until it's too late is that you are wiring your brain to experience pleasure and getting aroused under specific conditions.

• In porn, women are supposed to have great bodies saving you the time to go and look out for a real life potential partner and it just plain easier.

You get to experience the pleasure without any consequences; nobody 's getting pregnant, emotionally hurt; there 's no attachment whatsoever.

It's instantaneous with zero rejection except for you rejecting your behavior after watching it, and you might even maybe feel guilty-

• In porn you experience a vast amount of variety, you have countless videos to surfing for hours and hours and hours, to just keep yourself pleased and prevent you from getting bored.
It's been proven that men enjoy a wide variety of women in porn videos making it one of the main reasons many fall into the trap of this industry.

• Women are ideal for the porn industry that any guy would be able to find his heart's most beloved capricious desires there such as young women, older women Asian women, Latino, black, etc.

• It's always there for you, 24/7.

Technology got us big time on that one; nowadays it's much easier just to dump all of your negative feelings and just get to business no matter where you are or how late it is.

• It's certain to score in pornography; you experience certainty knowing your desires will be fulfilled and that you'll feel better. Everybody is happy, they all willingly have sex right away, fulfilling your ultimate fantasies of an easy score without any physical exhaustion or feedback from a partner.

• In real life, you don't have that. You're being brainwashed by the porn industry to believe the lies you see. I am willing to bet you, of all the things you see nowadays online, any significant potential partner you're looking for, would be nauseated by the thought of doing those things....

Chapter 5:

Is This really Worth it?

Before we get started, I'd like to challenge you in case you still t1'y rationalizing watching porn.

I challenge you to go 30 days without watching porn, if you manage to accomplish that then you're not addicted to porn in the short term, in the long run. It will get worse and I'd recommend getting rid of it as soon as possible, during these 30 days, you may please yourself as much as you want using ONLY your imagination or a partner!

No magazines, no sites and no photos! Brief consequences of watching porn:

• *Low on energy concentration and focus.*
Masturbating drains energy and burns lots of calories and with porn it's never enough, there will be times when you'll crave out of boredom, and it'll drain out your energy leaving you feeling helpless feeling like doing nothing and wondering what the heck just happened that day.

• *Wasting a heck load of time* browsing looking for perfection which does not exist, your brain becomes so adapted to find something better that you'll never settle for something. The process keeps getting longer and longer, consuming your time looking through categories with endless varieties and the next time you browse to find something you'd want something different, which takes, even more, time.

When you could be using it hanging out with friends, family, playing sports, study or improving yourself for a better future.

• *Experiencing no fulfillment* with your partner sexually or emotionally since you're exposing yourself to be aroused from other men / women which ends up wrecking your intimacy and destroying the marriage with your partner feeling rejected/hurt and possibly cheating on you to fill the gap or even worse, you wanting to experience somebody else and cheating on your partner whilst also finding that un-fulfilling.

That's because pornography also causes you to keep looking for a better-looking partner physically rather than balancing your choice based on significant factors such as mental attractiveness and compatibility, remember, sex is a way to connect intimately.

Chapter 6:

How it works in details

1. Dopamine &Addiction

In male subjects, there are five primary chemicals involved in sexual arousal and response and the one that plays the most significant role in pornography addiction is dopamine.

Dopamine plays an important part in the brain system that is responsible for reward-driven learning. Every type of reward that has been studied increases the level of dopamine transmission in the brain, and a variety of addictive drugs and stimulants such as cocaine, amphetamine, and methamphetamine, influence the dopamine system directly and cause a release. Dopamine surges when a person is exposed to novel stimuli, particularly if it is sexual, or when a stimulus is more arousing than anticipated. Since erotic imagery triggers more dopamine than sex with a close partner, exposure to pornography leads to an "arousal addiction" and teaches the brain to prefer the image and become less satisfied with real-life sexual partners, not to mention always browsing for more and more images.

2. The Coolidge effect & Variety

Why do men keep seeking out a new variety of sexual images rather than settling for satisfaction with the same ones?

The reason is attributed to the Coolidge effect, a phenomenon seen in mammalian species.

It's when males exhibit renewed sexual interest if introduced to new receptive sexual partners, even after turning down sex from former but still available sexual partners.

This neural mechanism is one of the primary reasons for the addiction to Internet pornography.

3. Sexually explicit material triggers mirroring neurons in the male brain.

These neurons, which are involved in the process for how to mimic & mirror a behavior, contain a system that correlates to a specific planning out of the conduct.

In the case, this mirror neuron system triggers an arousal, which leads to sexual tension and a need for an outlet. The reality is that when he acts out by masturbating, it leads to hormonal and neurological consequences, which are designed to bind him to the object he is focusing on.

Naturally it would be his wife, but for many men, it is an image on a screen.

Pornography thus enslaves countless viewers to an unrealistic picture, hijacking the biological response intended to bind a man to his wife and therefore inevitably loosening that bond.

4. *Dysfunctional satisfactory system & the journey to the pursuit of satisfaction*

Overstimulation of the reward system that occurs after repeated dopamine spikes as a result of viewing porn creates desensitization(numbing the receptors), which happens when dopamine receptors start malfunctioning after an overload of stimulating chemicals.

Then, as a result, the brain doesn't respond as much to pleasure so we feel less rewarded from the arousal which drives us to extend our search for satisfaction.

Leading to longer porn sessions and more porn viewing which spikes, even more, dopamine which causes, even more, numbness.

Conclusion of this chapter:

• Internet porn offers variety, novelty and constant renewal of fantasies; one can escalate both with more novel "partners" and by viewing new and unusual genres.

• There are almost no physical limitations to porn consumption making it an extremely dangerous activity to indulge in and waste your time.

• Unlike drugs and food, Internet porn doesn't eventually activate the brain's natural aversion system which forces you to stop.

• The age user's start watching porn is usually during teenage years when teen's brain is at its peak of dopamine production and neuroplasticity, making it highly vulnerable to addiction and rewiring.

Chapter 7:

How to Form Better Habits

You'll have to do the following in order to break free from this addiction:

• **Train your imagination to feel aroused by women you imagine, preferably a woman who is not a porn-star, rather look for a woman who fits your preference and choice.**

Practice closing your eyes and being intimate with that woman getting into the process of training yourself to be aroused without having to watch porn or look at photos.

It's paramount because you'll train your mind to be responsible for your arousal and it actually will help you controlling it in due time when it's needed.

• **Whenever you are aroused, get away from technology, and go to a private place to masturbate instead.**

It's extremely crucial since you WILL rationalize watching porn if you have a phone / PC/ tablet with you.

The key behind this is rigidly programming your mind to be in charge and control of such emotions and urges and their release.

You will notice a major difference within weeks of practicing this.

Grab a paper and pen and answer the following:

- Under which circumstances do you tend to watch porn?
- How do you rationalize the action?

You actually have inner conversations thorough the day without even noticing it!

What are the things you tell yourself right before watching porn that minimize the pain of watching it and maximize the pleasure?

• Under which emotional state do you watch porn?

• What can you do right now to avoid getting into such lousy states?

• What are the possible excuses you might come up with in the future to rationalize watching it?

• What are the statements you can tell yourself to keep yourself in alignment with your commitment you're making here to prevent you from falling off track? What can you tell yourself that would make you feel disgusted just by mentioning the word "porn"?

• What would you tell yourself when somebody tells you to take it easy on yourself?

• **Get into the mindset of looking for attractiveness into a**

relationship and not just physical attraction.

Write down on a paper:

- Why you want an intimate bond and why you will never settle for just mere physical attraction?
Anybody can be physically attracted, few can be mentally attracted and to be honest, a mental attraction is what keeps you going as the body ages.

- Why you'd rather suffer the massive amount of pain than compromise your values and watch porn?

• Read your answers and vows daily on a regular basis for at least one week until they are carved in your mind and you can rationalize them subconsciously anytime!

These are the exact steps I had to follow and justify for me to break free from watching porn. I wanted more out of life, and now I have more energy to get me through the day fully functioning, and I feel much better about myself since I am in alignment with my core values.

I hope you'll take action on all of the steps advised above!

I can show you the path; you have to walk it and take the steps!

Chapter 8:

Conclusion

If you find this book helpful and worth the value you've purchased it for, please do leave an accurate feedback of the book, this will help me improving the book, and it will reach more people as well as help others deciding whether they find it to be the right one for them.

I sincerely hope you'll take action on the instructions advised in the book as well as you sharing it with others who are struggling with this kind of addiction.

It's been an honorable journey serving you and providing you with what's necessary for you to grow and expand beyond your current limits and challenges.

Take action and live the life you truly deserve, it's simple, it's not easy changing your life, it takes dedication if you're meant to succeed, you will, because the mind translates your values and standards into a reality.

Huge Thank You and Words of Gratitude!

First and foremost, Thank You for downloading this book. At the end of the day, I'm extremely grateful for every download and every purchase. It makes me smile and motivates me. I wish that every person would put their best forward to the human race. I hope you unlimited mental strength and discipline to achieve your goals and dreams. Together we can make the difference.

If you found the information useful, I would be extremely grateful if you could write a short Amazon review. It does make the difference, and I read every review and take notes. I want to improve my books so that I can provide more value to other people. I know that my future books will give you the best experience possible

Copyright

Author: Daniel Rodgers

Publisher: Transcendence Publishing

Email: transpublishing@inbox.lv

Disclaimer